INDIUM

The

MISSING TRACE MINERAL

The newly discovered supplement for vibrant health

DR. ROBERT LYONS

INDIUM: The Missing Trace Mineral, The Newly Discovered Supplement for Vibrant Health.

By Dr. Robert Lyons

FIRST PRINTING
Copyright © 2001

New Health Press, Inc,
PO Box 530099,
Henderson, NV 89053-0099

IMPORTANT:

Table of Contents

INTRODUCTION

Indium, while not yet a house-hold word, will likely rocket skyward to that status within only weeks of you reading this book.

Only very rarely is a nutritional product discovered that has been found to have such wonderful bene-fits, and yet so little known, and not at all publicized.

Such is the case with the trace mineral, indium. First patented for nutritional use in 1980, its many users report life-changing benefits. Shared mainly by word-of-mouth among satisfied users, it's now time for the complete story of indium to be told.

Do you have a health problem that's plagued you for some time, without relief no matter what you've done? Do you need more energy, a slimmer, trimmer body, a more youthful appearance, stronger muscles or a host of other positive and healthful changes to your life?

All that and more may be easily within your grasp, utilizing the power of indium. Read on to discover the full benefits of this important trace mineral. Utilizing the latest cutting-edge research, and newly patented in 1999, indium can be added to your diet quickly and easily. But you must be sure you are getting the correct form of indium, and in the correct amount.

This is the only book that contains the precise information you need to experience the many advantages of indium.

DR. ROBERT LYONS
SEPTEMBER, 2001

CHAPTER 1

Trace Minerals and Good Health

People from the beginning of time have recognized the value of minerals. Many cultures used minerals to help relieve various health problems. The Chinese used seaweed, the Greeks used iron-enriched water, and the people of biblical times used salt as a purifying agent. It was not until the 19th century, however, that research and study of minerals began in a significant fashion. By the early 20th century, minerals had been recognized for their importance in human nutrition.[1]

Minerals are inorganic substances found in the soil and water. Plants are able to convert these inorganic minerals into organic ones. Humans eat the plants, and ingest second-stage organic minerals. Humans cannot assimilate inorganic minerals - they must be organic before they become bioavailable to our bodies. For this reason, some experts advocate drinking distilled water, as the body cannot use the inorganic dissolved minerals in spring or well water.[1]

Minerals help the structural components of the body. They also serve as catalysts that help regulate other bodily processes. In this regard, they are similar to enzymes in the body. It's been said for years that calcium helps make strong bones and teeth, while iron helps

Humans cannot assimilate inorganic minerals — they must be organic before they become bioavailable to our bodies.

make rich, red blood.[1] With minerals, man lives well. Without them, he does not.

Minerals act as either a major part of the chemical reaction, or a catalyst thereto. Suffice it to say that minerals, both macro- and micro-minerals, are required for human life. In fact, some minerals can be considered as substitutes for prescription drugs, lithium being the first mineral that comes to mind in this regard.

Throughout the ages of man's recorded history, minerals have been used for various health problems. At times, they were the only treatment available. Some of these uses for minerals included anemia, pica (mineral deficiency), dermatitis, skin diseases, epilepsy, tuberculosis, appetite rejuvenation, convulsions, rickets, premature gray hair, tooth problems, life extension, anti-parasitic, stomach problems, diphtheria, rheumatism, muscle pains, varicose veins, burns, gout, pleurisy, tumors, insanity, yellow fever, suicide, homicide and other criminal behavior. [2]

Of interest here is that indium, as demonstrated in a study by Dr. Henry Schroeder, helps the body absorb and use more of the other trace minerals than it would otherwise. Dr. Schroeder found that levels of copper and manganese in the kidneys were directly proportional to the ingestion of indium. [3, 4]

CHAPTER 2

The Hidden History of Indium

While indium has been used for years in the medical field, its widespread nutritional use is more recent.[5] The homeopathic remedy of Indium Metallicum has been used for perhaps seventy years or so for such problems as headache, migraine, backache, sneezing, acne, mouth sores, sore throat and other throat problems, productive cough, neck and shoulder stiffness and muscle pain.[6]

Another homeopathic reference lists dozens of uses for indium: depression, headache, lack of concentration, dizziness, eye pain, eye irritation, runny nose, sneezing, nasal congestion, sinus pressure, mouth sores, sore throat, mouth ulcers, lethargic appetite, nausea, bloated feeling in the stomach, abdominal pain, intestinal and bowel problems, urinary problems, trembling in hands and arms, fatigue in the legs, generalized pain throughout body, sleepiness in the afternoon, fever, weakness, irritability and menstrual problems.[7]

Originally patented in 1980, and newly patented in 1999, indium has been used effectively and safely by many sophisticated nutritional consumers. In fact, the 1999

patent specifically mentions that
the nutritional use of indium, when
done in accordance with the proper

---

*Testing done in 1975 was unable
to determine indium levels in the
body due to its low
concentration.*

---

formula and the proper type of
indium, meets the Food and Drug
Administration requirements for its
Generally Recognized As Safe des-
ignation.

The FDA's studies on indium
indicates that it would take 20,000
times more than that used for nutritional purposes to present a toxic
problem to the body. An entire bottle of liquid Indium-XL is less than

1/20th of the amount needed for such an overdose. Simply put, indium (in sulfate form) is a safe supplement to use for its many bene-

---

Indium exists in such small amounts, and is not water-soluble in nature, that it is simply not in the food chain.

---

fits. Dr. Henry Schroeder, whose work will be discussed at length in this book, found in his 1971 study that indium is non-toxic when taken orally at the recommended amounts.

Indium is a safe nutritional product for use by the public, you and I. [8] Having said that, let us discuss in detail the history of indium, specifically as it relates to its nutritional use. Much of the information that follows is taken from official documents on file in the U.S. Patent Office.

Indium occurs in very small amounts in the earth's crust. It is for this reason that it is designated a trace mineral, or as some call it, a micro-mineral. As you are aware, minerals, by their very nature, are inorganic. They cannot be utilized directly by the human body while in their inorganic form.

We need various minerals to live, the names with which we all are familiar: calcium, iron, copper, zinc and so on. But these minerals must be rendered organic if our bodies are to absorb them. We cannot chew on a penny and hope to get our daily supply of copper.

Most often, we receive our minerals from the foods we eat. Simply stated, plants absorb the inorganic minerals from the soil, and, through photosynthesis, convert them to an organic form that humans can use.

This is all well and good for minerals that exist in sufficient quantities in the soil. Indium, however, is in such small amounts, and is not water-soluble in nature, so that it is simply not in the food chain. Estimates place the level of indium in food at a maximum of .005 parts per million. Different estimates put the level of indium in the soil at either so low it can't be measured, or altogether non-existent.[2] Testing done in 1975 was unable to determine indium levels in the body due to its low concen-

Early on, it was found that if indium was to be of any value as a mineral supplement, it had to be made into the water-soluble sulfate form.

tration.[8] Whether it once existed in a water-soluble form and has been depleted from the farmland soil over the decades or whether plants are simply not able to convert it via photosynthesis is irrelevant. The fact remains that unless we supplement with indium, we simply will not have it in our diets — and we will lose its many benefits.

Notwithstanding this fact, one should not make the conclusion that, since we are ingesting little or no indium naturally, indium is not

---

The FDA's studies on indium indicates that it would take 20,000 times more than that used for nutritional purposes to present a toxic problem to the body

---

a mineral needed by the human body.

Rather, since we can live, albeit with disease and health problems, without indium, we must come to the following conclusion: indium is not required for life, but it is required for health!

One might appropriately ask, how could the beneficial properties of indium remain hidden from all the researchers for so long?

The answers lies in their flawed logic which ran something like this:

1) Since indium has never been found in a water-soluble compound, it cannot grow into vegetation, nor be found in meats, nor in any foods.
2) And, since it never shows up in complete autopsies,
3) Therefore, it is not necessary for life, so, therefore, it can not be needed for health.

We now know that this logic is seriously flawed because of the benefits that have been discovered in the past few years.

And since nearly all researchers passed by indium in their studies in favor of other trace minerals, we can surmise that had the research done on chromium, copper, zinc and the like been duplicated for indium, the results and benefits for indium would be even more outstanding, and much more publicized.

One thing is certain: if our intake of other trace minerals was reduced to .005 parts per million, we would see much greater sickness and disease. All this points to indium being vital for our continued good health, and a solution to some of mankind's most dreaded health problems.[9]

Early on, it was found that if indium was to be of any value as a mineral supplement, it had to be made into the water-soluble sulfate form. Additionally, even if made water-soluble, indium still binds with food in the stomach, rendering it useless. Indium is not absorbed by the body's digestive tract in the presence of food, as demonstrated in studies done in 1971 and 1973.[8]

Perhaps this is the reason that so many other nutritional researchers simply gave up on indium. Fortunately, one scientist doggedly continued his research until he found the answer.

Dr. Henry Schroeder was the scientist who conducted dozens upon dozens of experiments related to indium. Perhaps you have never heard of Dr. Schroeder, but you benefit from his research every day.

He is the man who pioneered the work on removing lead from gasoline. Without Dr. Schroeder's research on unleaded gasoline, our economies and financial lives would be at a standstill today.

Dr. Schroeder found that indium sulfate is hygroscopic, meaning that it absorbs water. Therefore, the only way that indium sulfate can be utilized as a nutritional supplement is in a liquid form. Indium pills or powder would absorb nine molecules of water for every molecule of indium, and quickly become waterlogged, as well as ruining the package in which it was placed.

Another scientist who devoted countless hours to the study of indium was Dr. Walter Mertz. Both Doctors Mertz and Schroeder have had portions of their significant life's work published in scholarly journals, such as Trace Elements in Human and Animal Nutrition, both the 4th and 5th editions.[10, 11]

All this points to indium being vital for our continued good health, and a solution to some of mankind's most dreaded health problems.

Dr. Mertz, of the Human Nutrition Research Center, U.S. Department of Agriculture, even edited the 5th edition, a further testimony to his professionalism and high regard by his peers. Dr. Schroeder published no less than thirteen studies on indium in peer review scientific journals, a high level of achievement by any standard.

CHAPTER 3

Indium and Cancer

While indium research is still ongoing, one interesting, and perhaps quite remarkable, situation has been uncovered. Indium is helping health problems in major ways that, until now, were considered beyond the scope of nutrition and/or modern medicine.

One of those health problems that indium may help is cancer. It has been shown to be effective against Walker 256 carcinosarcomas, and more research for its further use is ongoing.[13] In a more general fashion, a 1983 study found that indium sought out and saturated tumor tissue.[14] This is good news given the general tumor-reducing characteristics of indium.

Leading the field in indium and cancer research was Dr. Schroeder, mentioned at length earlier. His curiosity was initially aroused by indium in a 1971 study in which he found that indium supplementation caused a lower incidence of tumors.[15] This spurred him on to look further.

In this study, other rare earth minerals, such as scandium, gallium and palladium, all increased the rate of tumor incidence, some by nearly double. Only indium resulted in a lesser incidence of cancerous tumors, on average a 40% reduction. Schroeder also found that, as regards to lung cancer, indium was

A 1971 study found that indium supplementation caused a lower incidence of tumors.

highly anti-carcinogenic as compared to the other trace minerals, and performed better than the non-indium supplemented group.[16]

In one study, indium was found to inhibit the growth of both MCF-7 and HeLa human cervical malignant carcinoma cell lines.[13]

One interesting case is the use of the non-sulfate form of indium in the case of a man with a tumor of the rectum which had metastasized to his liver. Indium octreotide was used in this case, and, while not as potent as the sulfate form, resulted in a dramatic decrease in the size of the tumor and the disappearance of all symptoms.[13] One can only imagine what might have happened had indium sulfate been used.

There are rare cancers called thymomas. These tumors usually occur concurrent with thymus glandular problems, myasthenia gravis and various immune problems. This type of cancer is difficult to manage and treat. Discovered in its early stages, there is a reasonable likelihood of recovery. At later stages, due to much controversy regarding the proper treatment to use, a good outcome is much less likely. One patient given the octreotide form of indium had a successful outcome, opening the way for further study and use of indium against this cancer.[13]

Carcinoid tumors and pancreatic tumors have also been helped using indium octreotide. Three patients were in this study, and two of the three experienced very good improvement (tumors decreased by more than 50%). The study concluded that indium could be used in patients with neuroendocrine tumors.[13]

Indium and bone cancer has also been studied, and found to have positive benefits.[13]

In my limited experience with terminal cancer patients and indium supplementation, I have not found indium to be effective a changing the outcome. But, interestingly, among the noticeable benefits was in the area of comfort.

My patients all seem to have much reduced pain. Some were able to discontinue pain medication altogether, and some to reduce the medication significantly.

Also, their normally pale skin was replaced by a healthier-looking pink. They even reported feeling almost well. Unfortunately, for my patients at least, all ultimately succumbed to their cancers.

CHAPTER 4

Indium and Weight Loss

Dr. Henry Schroder's landmark work with indium also extends to the use of indium for weight loss. This was actually discovered in his 1971 study of indium and cancer.[16]

He found that the use of indium resulted in a lower body weight. This is likely accomplished via the "master feedback loop" which will be discussed further in Chapter 7. At even the lowest levels of supplementation, weight loss and/or lack of weight gain was noticed.[8]

Of even more interest is the fact that indium was more active in females than males. Since women have less muscle mass than men, indium may give them the extra boost they need to lose weight. Anecdotal reports by users indicate that both men and women experience the weight loss they desire, so perhaps this difference is only a scientific anomaly.

In the 1971 study, Dr. Schroeder graphed very interesting results. He found that, after maturity, females without indium added 20% of their weight on as fat, while those supplementing with indium added on no fat at all. He also discovered that those using indium

had better health than those without indium. For males, indium
helps maintain the muscle mass
normally lost to age-related
declines in growth hormone and
free testosterone. Thus, for both
male and female, indium results in
more stable weight throughout life,
without the ups and downs that
endanger our health.[16]

Thus, from all of the above we
can surmise that indium accom-
plishes weight loss in several different ways.

We know that indium has a
beneficial effect on the thyroid
gland. By potentiating this gland,
and helping support proper thyroid
levels, more calories are burned and
weight is normalized. I can recall
that perhaps more than thirty years

ago some health experts advocated using thyroid medications solely for their weight loss benefits. Indium is certainly a less expensive and more physiologically beneficial alternative.

Indium also provides an energy boost to most, if not all, people who supplement it to their diet. More energy usually results in more physical activity, thus providing a commensurate increase in calorie burning. Increased activity, over time, results in greater muscle mass. Since muscle tissues requires four times more calories to sustain itself than does fatty tissue, this raises the resting metabolic rate. Thus, even while sleeping, people burn more calories than their sedentary counterparts. While it may sound astounding, it is indeed possible to lose weight while you are sleeping. Proper attention to the metabolic rate will accomplish

---

Females without indium added 20% of their weight on as fat, while those supplementing with indium added on no fat at all.

---

that very benefit. Bodybuilders have known this fact for years. They work out for hours every day in order to strive to add pounds of muscle to their bodies. As a result, some of them need to eat thousands upon thousands of calories every day just to maintain bodily functions. For those of us not so inclined to work so hard and so long, indium supplementation provides much of the same benefits.

The implications of these findings are tremendously valuable for you and I. First, we should supplement with indium if only to receive its health benefits, quite apart from weight loss. For weight loss, indium may just be what we need to stop, and perhaps reverse, the age-related weight gain that comes on so easily and is so hard to lose. For those of us over 40 years of age, indium may make up for the normal decline of growth hormone, and perhaps even go beyond that, taking us to new levels of fitness, health and vibrant living.

Chapter 5

Indium and Increased Life Span

Americans rank 17th in life span when compared with other modern countries.[2] This is likely due in part to a decreased intake of important minerals, indium being the prime one for this discussion. Even more distressing is that man appears to be designed to live as long as 145 years.

We have known for years that a slightly lower calorie intake results in an increased life span. Dozens of scientific studies over the last two decades amply support this finding.

As discussed in Chapter 4, indium helps produce satisfactory weight loss in both men and women.

One of the ancillary findings of Dr. Schroeder's research is that indium appears to consolidate life expectancy.

Simply stated, this means that as we age, we will live more of our life span with a higher quality of life with indium than without indium. More research is needed specifically in this area, but the preliminary results are comforting. Imagine - we could live nearly all of our days energetic, vibrant, healthy and full-of-life. No more long stays in hospitals or nursing homes that characterize the last months or years of many people's lives.

CHAPTER 6

Indium and Improved Health

Indium has been found to cause an elevated mood and enhanced feeling of well-being in users. With the proliferation of medicines available for depression and related maladies today, indium may provide a more physiologic and certainly much less expensive alternative. Who among us has not had the occasional day when we felt a bit down, and not at our usual high level of physical strength or mental clarity? It is good to know that a simple drop of indium on the top of the tongue every morning propels us through life with vim and vigor, ready to meet and conquer each day's new challenges.

A May 11, 2000 press release from Reuter's Health network discusses the use of Substance P, an amino acid brain chemical, in helping depression, anxiety, stress and chemical addictions.[17] Substance P is thought by some to contain indium, thus explaining its positive benefits. Dr. Hunt, a London researcher, studied the use of Substance P in drug addictions, and found that it could be beneficial for those desiring to discontinue their drug use.[18] This confirms the anecdotal reports by indium users that alcohol and drug use were much easier to control or stop after taking a proper indium supplement. Dr. Hunt further stated that Substance P may be as effective as Prozac, a drug normally prescribed for depression.[18] Indium users have known of this benefit for over two decades now, with indium producing a feeling of well-being and euphoria after only a few days of use.

Eyeball pressure goes up from childhood from near 8/8, to teen numbers in the teens, and near 20/20 in senior years. An eye examination involves recording of the eye pressure on the person's record. At 20/20 the doctor is alerted, and at 25/25 he prescribes medication, which may have side effects. With enough indium, it has been reported that the numbers come down in a few months by 10-35% into a safer range.[12]

Persons with high blood pressure, such as over 160, will likely see it come down with enough indium. Dr. Walter Mertz, co-discoverer of the human need for chromium and retired head of the Human Nutrition branch of the Department of Agriculture, explained that chromium helps lower blood pressure, but the absorption of chromium is very poor. It is suggested that, in high blood pressure, both indium upon arising and chromium with a meal will be most effective in reducing blood pressure by about 15 points per month, to below 130. Meanwhile, a too low blood pressure will rise slowly, to over 100.

The mechanism for this action seems to be the ability of the indium to cause the body to absorb and use more of the chromium in the

Indium users have known of it's anti-depressant activity for over two decades now, with indium producing a feeling of well-being and euphoria after only a few days of use.

diet.[12] Interestingly, indium also seems to help the body recycle trace elements from the fluids in the large intestine. This is helpful to the body as the trace minerals are necessary for any number of physiological processes. Accordingly, this may account for the claims of health improvement for which there is no other satisfactory explanation.[19]

Indium increases the uptake of chromium in to the spleen by 90%, the lungs by 112%, the liver by 232%, the heart by 536% and the kidneys by 694%.[20]

Some of the most exciting research with indium relates to its use against pain and inflammatory processes, such as arthritis and similar problems. The previously mentioned chemical called Substance P is an amino acid that may contain indium, and plays an important part in relieving pain. One study tested it, and found that in eight of the patients, substance P was observed in the thymus gland. Additionally, Substance P travelled to sites of inflammation caused by various health problems. Certainly more research is required, but these results are very promising.[13]

Type Two diabetics using insulin may need to adjust their daily insulin because indium can change the need for insulin, sometimes occurring on the very first day of indium intake. An 80% reduction has been reported in as little as one week. Some diabetics have eliminated their need for insulin after several weeks of indium supplementation. While the mechanism for this is unclear, it may be that indium prompts the glandular complex to send more accurate signals to the pancreas, thereby resulting in a more stable level of insulin being secreted. Such diabetics need to keep both indium and insulin on hand for their needs. Of course, such an individual must monitor their blood sugar closely, either using the

---

Two major effects that indium has are in its ability to help the body assimilate other important nutrients and in increasing the life span of red blood cells from 90 to 120 days.

---

home testing kits, or by using a qualified health care provider.

Pregnant women's bodies use insulin to produce the hormone relaxin. Relaxin moves the baby into the optimum support position, thus preventing some premature deliveries. Relaxin later causes the pelvic area to become very elastic, helping a more comfortable and speedier delivery. Indium appears to help generate both insulin and relaxin in pregnant women.[12]

A very recent study with indium was conducted in Bat Ischl, Austria at the TCM Academy on patients suffering with Alzheimer's and Morbus Parkinson's disease. An oral application of Indium was used with 24 subjects using a double blind study in collaboration with the Austrian Morbus Alzheimer Society, M.A.S.

The protocol for both the control group and the test subjects included 1/2 hour per day of classical music, use of some specific

Chinese herbs, and massage therapy. Diet was not controlled.

The test subjects also received a daily drop of indium. The control group not using indium showed an overall improvement of 8% after 30 days. The indium group showed a 37% improvement in the same time period.

Improvements included more normal patient behavior, an improvement in stamina, better short term memory and some of the very dependent patients returned to a significant level of self care.

The Academy was so impressed, that at the time of the writing of this book, they are in the midst of a second study.

The indicators of the effectiveness of the amounts of indium intake and absorption are return to normal range of libido in both men and women in two weeks, a powerful sense of well-being overtakes the user within one to two weeks, physical energy and strength increases within two weeks, families report that the user is "easier to live with," the sense of smell returns, less sleep is needed within one to two weeks, type two diabetic use of insulin may decline within two weeks, glaucomic-type eye pressure is reduced within three months.

Most of the benefits of indium occur within 5-10 days of supplementation. Some serious health problems, such as blood sugar imbalances, neurological problems and eye problems take two to three

weeks to see good benefits. More
serious health issues may take up to
6 months to see improvement, but
even that is better than the hope-
lessness offered by other alterna-
tives.

CHAPTER 7

Indium and Glandular Health

Indium appears to work via a hypothalamus feedback loop complex in the human body. Apparently, this is the mechanism that causes indium users to experience a recognizable feeling of euphoria and well-being. These benefits could be either from particular glands or from the "Master Gland" (pituitary) feedback control system, which controls production of at least thirty-one hormones. Such production is regulated by the hypothalamus (Master Gland) feedback loop, which responds several times per minute.[12]

As mentioned earlier, Substance P is a fairly new amino acid-type substance, and may indeed contain indium. Men have more Substance P than women, and this may be what largely protects men from having thyroid problems to the extent that women normally do. A 1986 study by O.R. Tumilasci and his team found that the thyroid gland showed a sensitivity to Substance P. [21]

Thyroid associated opthalmopathy is an inflammatory eye problem related to Grave's Disease and Thyroid Eye Disease (TED). Indium has been used in these cases as a standard tool for medical diagnosis. The form of indium used, In111, is designed solely as a diagnostic tool and not a treatment. Interestingly, some patients report a lessening of the symptoms after this medical diagnostic test using indium, even though the indium is in the octreotide and not the sulfate form. One researcher found that the indium is absorbed by the thyroid and the lymphocytes at the back of the eye. His conclusion is that these areas of the body are indium-deficient, and the indium most readily floods to those sites. Another study involving the non-sulfate form of indium sought to determine the octreotide's effect on thyroid eye disease. In this study, 24% of the participants experienced improvement after the indium treatment.[13]

This researcher went on to discuss a very interesting hypothesis.

He believes that cadmium is a toxic metal which helps cause Grave's Disease and TED. Cadmium is introduced into the body via smoking tobacco, high levels of estrogen (women), and eating higher amounts of leafy green vegetables. Cadmium is number 48 on the element chart, indium is number 49. He believes that elements next to each other in the elemental table are highly antagonistic to each other. Thus, the cadmium levels are depleting what little, if any, indium is in the body. When indium is added to the diet, it becomes antagonistic to the cadmium, flushes it out of the body, and restores health to the eye.[13]

Chapter 8

Indium and Sports Performance

The strenuous exerciser, who normally stops exercising due to muscular pain, should be able to increase their workouts by 10% without pain. Indium helps reduce the painful buildup of lactic acid by removing it more quickly from the tissues.[12]

One interesting but anecdotal story of the use of indium relates to the owner of a racing horse. After retiring the horse from a successful racing career, the owner supplemented the horse's feed with indium for two weeks. Immediately thereafter, the old horse ran in six races, winning all six and setting two new track records.[22]

Other anecdotal reports indicate that indium helps with any exercise routine. Some reports mention an even greater benefit for those over 40 than those under 30. This seems reasonable given that age-related decline in almost all hormonal substances in the body begins in the 30s, and perhaps the effect of these decreased hormones is felt more strongly after 40 years of age.

Even so, a study performed in Budapest, Hungary which should be published in a prominent, peer review journal in the coming months, demonstrated that even 20 to 30 years olds can benefit from indium supplementation.

The study was conducted using 15 male subjects who were all members of Hungary's National Kung Fu Championship Team.

Blood work showed all subjects to be free from parasites and disease. Then each one was measured for stamina.

For 60 days, each subject was given one drop of indium on the tongue per day on an empty stomach.

After 60 days, all were retested. Thirteen out of 15 showed 20% improvement in overall stamina and no side effects were noted by any of the subjects.

Two of my patients in their late thirties and early forties are long distance runners so I tried an experiment with them. They each took one drop of indium per day for two weeks.

After two weeks, they both reported that they were able to run about 30% farther.

Two of my body builder friends took indium as their sole supplement and ate regular food for 90 days. After two months, they were able to bench press 40% more weight.

NOTE OF CAUTION:

Athletes should not supplement with creatine while taking indium. Indium has been shown to increase the uptake of creatine in the blood over 500%. This level of creatine in the blood could pose a serious health risk.

CHAPTER 9

Getting the Most from Indium Supplementation

For good reasons, correcting an indium shortage appears to be more dramatic than that of any other trace element. Our intake of other trace elements can never get anywhere close to zero without endangering our lives.

Not so with indium. Indium intake is at zero in the non-supplementing population.

So the benefits of taking indium, at a 100% level, become very obvious just by looking at the average person over 40 in our modern society.

Most do not get fully restorative sleep. They just don't feel good. Their memory could be better. High blood pressure is killing them with strokes and heart attacks. They have a whole host of hormone problems. They have a problem absorbing other trace elements into their vital organs, like the heart, brain, liver, kidneys and spleen.

We all need indium, but we cannot get it in our food. We can't even rush down to the store to buy some. In addition, over the years, researchers have determined several difficulties in creating a viable indium supplement (see Table 9-1).

Using the preparation and delivery system covered by a U.S. Patent, EPR,LLC, has been able to

---

TABLE 9-1

Difficulties in Creating a Viable Indium Supplement.

- Indium is not present in any of the food we eat.

- Indium is not bioavailable in the natural inorganic form.

- Organic indium rapidly binds to food in the digestive system rendering it useless.

- Solid organic indium is so hygroscopic that it absorbs massive amounts of water making it impossible to produce in pill or capsule form.

- The presence of other minerals "rob" the receptor sites necessary for proper uptake of indium.

- Most organic indium compounds are not soluble in water.

---

get around all of the obstacles encountered by earlier researchers.

A normal day's amount of indium is 10 milligrams. Most of the indium will be absorbed in the mouth and stomach.

It is for this reason that indium supplementation must be done at such time as there is little or no food in the stomach. This is accomplished quite easily by taking one drop of indium on top of the tongue immediately upon arising in the morning.

An informal testing of the benefits of indium involves being aware of the sense of well-being, or joy of living, which arises in less than a week after beginning supplementation. Temporarily discontinuing the use of indium will indicate

the optimal level of supplementation for that individual.

If the sense of well-being disappears after about four days, then

---

TABLE 9-2

Tips for Proper Indium
Supplementation

• Take in the liquid indium sulfate
  form — 10 mg per drop.

• Start with one drop per day. Use
  tests in Table 9-3 to determine
  optimum amount.

• Place the drop of indium on the top
  of the tongue after at least 8 hours
  without food — preferably upon
  first arising from sleep and before
  putting anything in your mouth.

• Avoid eating or drinking for about
  30 minutes after application.

the level of indium is correct. If this feeling disappears after less than four days, the amount of indium taken can be increased slightly.

If the feeling lasts longer than four days, some indium is being wasted and the amount can be reduced slightly.[12]

In some cases, people have not noticed any significant change. Those individuals seem to fall into three different categories.

One group that fails to notice improvement with indium supplementation is the group of people, usually over 50, who have certain mineral deficiencies. These folks usually have a myriad of symptoms and ill health as a result of their deficiencies.

Levels of the essential minerals should be tested by health professionals. They can recommend spe-

---

TABLE 9-3

How to Monitor the Results of Indium Supplimentation

1. Prior to any supplementation, take note of how you feel and of how many hours of sleep you require each night to feel rested.

2. Take one drop of indium sulfate each morning (see Table 9-2) for about 30 days.

3. At the end of 30 days, note how you feel and how many hours of sleep you require each night to feel rested. (compare with Step 1.)

4. Note how long it takes for your sense of well-being to diminish. If it is less than four days, you can increase to two drops, if it is longer than 4 days, you may be able to reduce to one drop every other day.

cific supplementation for the minerals that are missing.

The second group that fails to notice significant improvement is the younger, healthier people who haven't yet been affected by the decreasing hormone output that seems to accompany aging.

This does not mean that these individuals cannot or are not benefiting. In this case the old adage, an ounce of prevention is worth a pound of cure is certainly applicable.

The third group, and perhaps the biggest one, are the people who have weakened immune systems. When the immune system is taxed, nothing works optimally — including the utilization of nutrients.

By far and away the best remedy that I know for this problem is
East Park's patented olive leaf
extract called *d*-Lenolate.™

TABLE 9-4

Reasons Why Indium Supplementation May Not Produce Noticeable Benefits

- Improper utilization. See Table 9-2.

- A deficiency in one or more important minerals. (Lots of other health problems would indicate this condition.) See a competent health professional for testing.

- A weakened immune system due to presence of pathogens and parasites. Supplement with *d*-Lenolate.™

- Endocrine system has not yet begun to demonstrate the slowing down due to aging. You may want to use indium as a preventative measure.

Without getting into the mechanisms of how d-Lenolate works, suffice it to say, that I have seen, first hand, the wonderful results.

Strengthening the immune system is very important. Maybe more so than the vast majority of people (including physicians) realize.

You see, drugs do not "cure" any disease. Herbs don't "cure" any disease. Vitamins and minerals do not "cure" any disease.

The only thing that cures disease in humans is the human immune system.

I am not suggesting that wholesome food, vitamins, minerals, herbs, and even drugs do not have a place, but when the immune system is burdened with pathogens and parasites, it needs help from a and parasites, it needs help from a anti-fungal, anti-bacterial, anti-viral, anti-parasitic supplement like d-Lenolate.™

Finally, the indium user should also note how long he sleeps, on average, before taking indium. It would be helpful to record the length of sleep time when awakening naturally without any outward signal. The indium user will most likely find that he sleeps less time each night, yet with the same feeling of energy and vitality upon arising. Most users report needing an hour or more less sleep per night. Users who must awake with an alarm for their daily duties will find that the same amount of sleep now results in a greater feeling of restfulness.[12]

Many changes are going to come about by our daily intake of indium. As you begin your supplementation program, note the positive (and negative — if any) changes that you experience along the way.

And, by all means, if you have serious medical conditions, consult a physician before you begin any and all supplementation or exercise programs.

Answers to Frequent Questions about Indium

Q. How does indium taste?

A. It has a clean, strong tart taste. You will be able to taste it, even one drop on the tongue. A phrase typically used is that it Tastes Terribly Tart While Working Wonderfully Well.

Q. Is indium safe?

A. Yes. Tests on animals show that it would have to be 1,000 times stronger to make a mouse sick. Most other trace elements are not that safe.

Q. What do I do if my child drinks

the entire bottle?

A. Is is so very tart that they are most likely unable to swallow a second time. Expect them to vomit. Have them eat any foods and drinks which they like, but not an excess amount. The emergency room could pump their stomach. In the indium contacting food, most of it will no longer be soluble in water, and will not be absorbed.

Q. How fast does it work?

A. It starts affecting glands the first day, but most new user benefits take over a week to reach a noticeable level.

Q. How do I get the most benefits?

A. By taking indium only upon arising, before brushing teeth, with no other food, drink or medicine in the mouth for at least ten minutes after   taking   the   indium. Undigested food in the stomach may compound with indium, rendering it useless, thus the need not to eat right before bedtime.

Q. What benefits can I expect from indium supplementation?

A. Long term reduction of rates and appearances of aging. A better immune system, reducing the severity and duration of colds, bruises and healing. Faster memory, less sleep, enhanced sense of well-being replacing depression, and much more.

Q. What is indium?

A. Element #49, indium, is never found as a water-soluble compound, so it is never in any food, or our bodies. It is about the tenth most scarce of all available elements. On the Periodic Table of the Elements, Indium connects the two largest groups of elements known to be useful to mammal nutrition. Thus, it becomes a true "missing link."

Q. How pure is indium?

It is 99.99% pure. Few other nutritional compounds are this pure.

Q. What is indium?

A. It is a soft mineral that never dissolves in water, until compounded by man. It is the third heaviest molecular element known to be useful in nutrition.

Q. Are there any precautions or contraindications?

A. Indium is not for use on broken skin, or in the eyes. It may have no benefits for Type One diabetics. The very low thyroid condition may correct too fast, producing a unique pressure headache. This is noticeable only upon awakening and is relieved by any activity. Stop intake until cleared, then try taking indium one day a week, then two days apart, three days and so on. Expect gradual disappearances of dry skin, dry hair, fatigue, anemia, bowel problems, irritability and poor physical strength. Also expect gradual benefits of weight loss, less sleep and more energy. This may take as long as 4 months, as the life cycle of red blood cells is about 120 days.

A source of iodine is essential in the diet. Morton Lite salt is especially effective in supplying needed iodine and rejecting excess water. Historically "Long term normalized thyroid is among the greatest of needed improvements in lifestyle known to medicine." Older people are slowest to respond, but the effort is well worth it. Be patient. Note: Headaches upon arising are a sign that the indium use is proceeding too fast, for that person. Take less indium for a short time.

Q. Will indium make me stronger?

A. Not directly. But you will be able

to extend your limit of activity as the indium hastens the removal of lactic acid. Thus, pain during exercise will be lessened, and you can work harder.

Timetable to See Benefits from Indium Supplementation

With recommended use, one can expect to see benefits from indium supplementation very quickly. The following chart lists the time frame in which some actual indium users saw positive benefits. Note: Individuals with serious illness and/or weakened immune systems typically see results after a longer time — depending on the seriousness of their conditions.

TIME	*POSITIVE BENEFIT*
1 Hour	*Sore throats stopped by spraying*

TIME	*POSITIVE BENEFIT*
2 Days	Less sleep needed
1 Week	Better comfort by ill people
1 Week	Sense of well-being
1 Week	Healing time of scratches, burns and bruises decreased
1 Week	Elimination of localized cancer pain
1 Week	Taste sensitivity restored in elderly
1 Week	Sense of smell regained
10 Days	Physical endurance increased
2 Weeks	Normalization of low blood sugar
2 Weeks	Hypoglycemia reduced to near normal
2 Weeks	Routine migraine headaches stopped - some cases in as little as a few hours
2 Weeks	Person with Parkinson's walks and talks better

TIME	*POSITIVE BENEFIT*
2 Weeks	*Normalization of saliva flow*
2 Weeks	*HIV/AIDS patients helped with diarrhea*
2 Weeks	*Libido returned to normal - for both male and female*
3 Weeks	*Eye pain disappears*
Few Weeks	*Diabetic control of sugar level*
2 Months	*Low blood pressure helped*
2 Months	*Menstrual cycle irregularity helped*
Few Mos.	*Eye pressure, glaucoma normalized - gradually*
Several Months	*Intestinal and bowel problems helped*
Several Months	*Hair growth returned*
Several Months	*High blood pressure helped - gradually*
Several Months	*Dry skin softened*

The Mysteries of Nutritional Indium, Element #49

Indium is a soft metal, which, on The Periodic Table of the Elements, joins the two largest groups of nutritional elements on that Table.

All the elements that we need for nutrition are listed as various numbers from number 1 to number 53. There are two groups of nutritional elements within these numbers. Indium, as number 49, joins these two groups of nutrients into one large group. Indium, Number

49, is a missing link, and a very important nutrient, that has been missing from our diet.

Indium has been discovered to be a needed element in the avoidance of many afflictions, and in achieving and maintaining a healthy condition. Previously, our attempts to correct these health afflictions have at times been met with unsatisfactory results, or even failure.

Just as with any other nutritional trace elements, the shortage symptoms of this newly discovered nutritional element are not "diseases." They are "deficiency symptoms." When we are short of iron or copper or zinc, only supplementing that particular element will correct our affliction.

Thus, to correct our indium deficiency, and restore our good health, all of us need to supplement with nutritional indium.

Based on extensive laboratory studies by Dr. Henry Schroeder, of seven rare earth trace minerals, six raised the cancer rates, and only indium is non-carcinogenic.

Another researcher, George Bonadio, sorted through volumes of data and determined that subjects taking indium have 26% less cancer and 46% fewer malignant tumors than non-indium users. [23]

In one of Bonadio's many papers concerning the subject of indium, he concludes:

> There are over forty reported benefits from indium. None of them can be corrected satisfacto-

rily by medicine, other nutrients, skilled treatment, proce-
dure or health care. They can
only be resolved by using indium! Thus, it follows that indium
is another nutritional trace element that is needed for many
areas of health. Many of the
benefits are associated with a
tighter control of glands and
hormones by the thyroid, working with the hypothalamus, reg-
ulating about 31 hormones. This
is a continuous correction. It
cannot be duplicated by a slow
dissolving pill of one or even
two dozen hormones. The half-
lives of 29 of our hormones
average to 30 minutes. Nine of
those hormones average at only
ten minutes. There is no way to
supplement these hormones by
any convenient commercial
means. [23]

Anecdotal Reports: Results from Indium Use

IMPORTANT NOTE: ANECDOTAL REPORTS ARE NOT VALID FOR MAKING SCIENTIFIC OR CATEGORICAL STATEMENTS ABOUT THE EFFICACY OF ANY SUBSTANCE. THESE ACCOUNTS HAVE BEEN TAKEN FROM UNSOLICITED LETTERS AND COMMENTS WHO HAVE USED EAST PARK RESEARCH, INC.'S INDIUM PRODUCT.

Anecdotal evidence from indium users has demonstrated the following results after a daily or two to three times per week supplementation schedule:

- High PSA, indicating prostate problems, dropped 75%.
- One doctor reports that some diabetic patients reduced their insulin intake by 80%.
- Parkinson's Disease sufferer reported improvement in walking and speech in two weeks.

- Numerous reports of helping the monthly menstrual cycle.
- Doctor reports two patients with HIV/AIDS improved in only two weeks.
- Increased dental health and longer times between routine teeth cleanings.
- Increase in mental energy and concentration.
- Two reports showing improvement in birthing children.
- Glaucomic eye pressure decreased without use of medication.
- Sports endurance and strength increased within ten days.
- Increased physical energy.
- Decrease in recurrent migraine headaches.
- More restful sleep, users may need an hour or more less sleep per night with increased energy.
- Memory improves.

- Hormone imbalances restored to normal.
- Other trace minerals become better absorbed by the body, for optimal nutrition.
- Improved immunity against colds and flu.
- Normalization of blood sugar levels.
- Improved prostate gland health.
- Improved thyroid health.
- Cuts, wounds, scratches and bruises heal easier and quicker.
- Habits of over-drinking and smoking more easily controlled.
- Potential life extension capabilities.
- Thins blood thereby reducing the risk of stroke by up to 60%.
- Reduces symptoms of menopause.
- Extends the lifetime of red blood cells.

- Assists in restoring youthful hair
  color and growth.

REFERENCES

1. Concoby, Robert H., "Discovered: Nature's Secret Fountains of Youth", Hanford Press, 1993.
2. Wallach, Dr. Joel, "Rare Earths: Forbidden Cures", DH Publishing Company, November 1994
3. Schroeder, Dr. Henry, "Interactions of Trace Metals in Mouse and Rat Tissues; Zinc, Chromium, Copper and Manganese with 13 Other Elements" in "Interactions of trace metals in rat tissues: Cadmium and nickel with zinc, chromium, copper, manganese", Journal of Nutrition 104: 167-168.
4. Schroeder, Dr. Henry, Journal of Nutrition 106:198-203, 1976.
5. Webster, W.B., "Pharmacokinetic and Biologic Distribution Studies of

Indium 111-Labeled Monoclonal Antibodies", New Perspectives in Cancer Diagnosis and Management 1(2):42-47, as reported in OncoLink, August, 2001.

6. Boericke, Dr. W., "Manual of Homoepathic Materia Medica", B. Jain Publishers, New Delhi, June, 1927.

7. Allen, Dr. Timothy, "The Encyclopedia of Pure Materia Medica", Medi-T, June, 2001.

8. Smith, Ivan C. et al, "Trace Metals in the Environment, Volume 5 - Indium", Ann Arbor Science Publishers, 1978.

9. Unattributed article, "Indium Is Just Plain Unbelievable, Like All Advances For Humans".

10. Underwood, Eric, editor, "Trace Elements in Human and Animal Nutrition, 4th Edition", Academic Press, New York, 1977.

11. Mertz, Walter, editor, "Trace Elements in Human and Animal Nutrition, 5th edition", Academic Press, New York, 1986.

12. Bonadio, George, "Methods for Administering Nutritional Indium", United States Patent, Washington, D.C., December 1999.

13. Unattributed article, "Indium", Internet file indium1.htm, June 20, 2001.

14. Southern, L.L., Journal of Nutrition 113(3): 688-96, March 19983.

15. Schroeder, Dr. Henry, Journal of Nutrition 101: 1431-8, 1971, as reported in "Trace Elements in Human and Animal Nutrition, 5th edition", 1986.

16. Schroeder, Dr. Henry, "Scandium, Chromium (VI), Gallium, Yttrium, Rhodium, Palladium, Indium in Mice: Effects on Growth and Life Span", Journal of Nutrition 101: 1431-8, 1971.

17. Reuters Health, "Brain Chemical Shows Way To New Drug Treatments", Reuter's Information Services, May, 2000.

18. Hunt, Stephen P., Nature 2000 405:180-83, May, 2000.

19. Unattributed article, "The Mysteries of Nutritional Indium, Element #49".

20. Lyons, Dr. Robert, letter dated November 14, 2000.

21. Tumilasci, O.R., "Influence of thyroid function upon 'Substance P' induced secretion of saliva by submaxillary glands", Hormonal Metabolic Research 18(4):234-7, April 1986.

22. Bonadio, George, "The Missing Link Nutritional Trace Element Has Been Found, and It Is Impressive", Watertown, NY, 2000.

23. Bonadio, George, "How Would It Be If We Found a New Nutritional Trace Element Needed for Life or Health?", Watertown, NY, 2000.